RETURNED

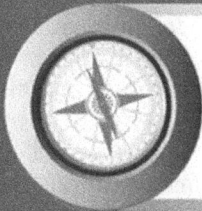

Missionary
Handbook
(Of Intimacy)

I0115623

By Dr. Adam Andeeve, PHD

Published by Easy Publishing Company
http://www.easypublishingcompany.com
contact@easypublishingcompany.com
Salt Lake City, UT 84108

ISBN-13: 978-0692228081
ISBN-10: 069222808X

First Edition: June 2013
Printed in the United States of America

Table of Contents

Introduction

"Men and women compliment each other not only physically, but also emotionally and spiritually... men and women have different strengths and weaknesses, and marriage is a synergistic relationship in which spiritual growth is enhanced because of the differences."
~Elder Merrill J. Bateman

I am writing this book because I feel like there is a tremendous need for the education of returned missionaries in the field of intimacy. Intimacy is one of those things that most parents don't want to worry about and most kids don't want to talk to their parents about. There has always been a fair amount of controversy surrounding this topic in the church. Some youth leaders try to teach this subject, but there are so many myths and misconceptions about intimacy that this may do more damage than help. Many leaders haven't even mastered this subject themselves, thus teaching incorrect beliefs and behaviors. But this book isn't sex education for kids. It's meant for adults and it's meant to guide these adults as they wade into previously unknown waters.

I wish that this book had existed when I had got back from my mission. I paid close attention during both health classes that I was required to take in school and felt like I knew all about the female genitals and exactly what happened during sex. It was my friends and the brief sex scenes I had seen on TV that taught me everything I knew. But both my friends and television turned out to be terrible teachers that horribly misrepresented sex and intimacy. My friends, the self-appointed "experts", were completely wrong about most of their claims and the sex scenes on TV were not accurate representations of real-life sex.

This book is perfect for anybody that is dating with the goal of looking for an eternal companion. I am writing this book primarily for men that belong to the Church of Jesus Christ of Latter Day Saints. However, I feel that the information herein can be informative and helpful to any person belonging to any other religion. Also, I feel like this can be a very informative book for women as well. I am a guy and I have several guy friends. We have had several discussions about our misconceptions about sex and intimacy. Since getting married, we have talked for hours about things we wish we would have known before we got married. I have talked with several couples about intimacy and had the idea to write a short, simple book that will cover the main things that most people don't know.

This book is perfect for those just finishing up their missions. It is good for those that have been home from their mission for a while and are dating. It is great for those that have recently gotten engaged and are getting ready for marriage. It would be a great gift for a girl to give to her husband or fiancé so that he may better understand how she works.

Note: This book deals with a very sacred and mature subject matter. At no time during the book am I trying to be crude or insensitive. However, I will be very straightforward and will not use slang terms. Sex and intimacy are ordained and encouraged by our Heavenly Father and have been advocated by every prophet in our dispensation.

Right off your Mission

"Love is like a flower, and, like the body, it needs constant feeding. The mortal body would soon be emaciated and die if there were not frequent feedings. The tender flower would wither and die without food and water. And so love, also, cannot be expected to last forever unless it is continually fed with portions of love, the manifestation of esteem and admiration, the expressions of gratitude, and the consideration of unselfishness."
~President Spencer W. Kimball

A simple way to tell how well a missionary has served the Lord his how apprehensive he or she is around the opposite sex when they first return home. If they have been serving the Lord with their whole heart, might, mind, and strength, then they will not have had time to think romantically about members of the opposite sex. Not even thinking about girls for a significant amount of time, most missionaries return home and are awkward around girls for at least a few weeks.

One of the most important recommendations I give to returned missionaries is to make a "spouse list" as soon as they can when they get off their mission. Do this while you are still so close to the spirit and before you have been exposed to all the worldly things. Take a healthy amount of time to read the scriptures, pray, and make a list of the traits that you feel would be important in a spouse. Separate your list out into categories that include spiritual, mental, physical, emotional, social, and sexual. Write as much as you can into these different categories and give them a ranking according to importance. Obviously, you won't find a girl that is perfect in every single category, but this list will help you steer clear of those that aren't even close.

Many missionaries think that they need to jump right back into the dating scene where they left off and "fill their canteen" to "make up for lost time." I recommend that you take your time and start the whole dating process over again. Just as you haven't had any dating experience for the past two years, you also haven't had to resist much sexual temptations for the past two years either. Getting into a tempting situation too soon can be difficult to overcome and dangerous. Ease into dating at a pace that feels most comfortable for you.

An easy way to get back into dating is to start off by spending time with female members of your family. Hang out with your mom, sisters, or female cousins until you feel comfortable around them. Try to make small talk with girls everywhere you go. Talk to them about the weather, current events, or their likes and dislikes. This exercise will help you feel much more comfortable around all girls and prepare you for your first date.

Your first date

"The most important meeting of the week is sacrament meeting, and the second most important is date night. I do believe it is very important that you put first on your calendar, after sacrament meeting, time together as husband and wife."
~Elder L. Tom Perry

My first (and possibly most important) recommendation for your first date is to go on a group date. That means that you need to be with at least one other couple. Like I mentioned earlier, you haven't been courting girls (hopefully) for quite a while. No matter how confident you feel, having another couple with you can take off quite a bit of pressure from the date in several different ways:

1- More people to create talking points
2- You have a wing man to help if you mess anything up
3- You have two people who are rooting for you to succeed. They can offer suggestions that you might need.
4- They won't leave you alone thus you won't need to worry as much about the physical aspect of dating.
5- Having another female along can make it more comfortable for your date. The girl you ask is probably more nervous about being your first date since your mission than you are.

Unlike other dates you may have been on before you mission, I recommend that you do some preparation before the date arrives. Think of things that you can talk about that might be fun for both you and your date. No matter how meaningful and life-changing your mission was, your date isn't interested in talking about it for the entire date. Make a small cheat sheet of items that would be fun to talk about on the date and keep it in your pocket. Do your best to limit yourself to 2 topics that start with "On my mission..."

Pick a date activity that is simple, but not thoughtless. For example, bowling is simple, but it is also thoughtless. You didn't have to do much thinking to figure out what to do for bowling. A hike, on the other hand, may be simple but also takes planning. You have to choose the hiking trail and plan it out. Do something that you like to do and that will give you plenty of time to talk and get to know each other.

Refrain from 'all-day dates.' This is especially true for your very first date, but it is also a good idea for any other 'first dates' you may have in your life. Keep it under 2-3 hours. This way, if the date isn't going well, you and your date don't have to endure through a bad time just because you promised her a 5-hour date. If the date goes well, you will leave her happy and wanting more.

Hopefully I haven't scared you out of dating. As long as you are prepared and don't worry too much, everything will go just fine. You have just returned from selling people on a book that they didn't think they wanted. Now you are on a date with a girl who is obviously interested enough to say yes to a date with you. This should be a piece of cake!

Your first girlfriend

"Soul mates" are fiction and an illusion; and while every young man and young woman will seek with all diligence and prayerfulness to find a mate with whom life can be most compatible and beautiful, yet it is certain that almost any good man and any good woman can have happiness and a successful marriage if both are willing to pay the price.
~BYU Devotional

After a good amount of dating you will probably find a girl that you like a little bit more than the rest of the girls. If you've only dated one girl, you really don't know if you want her as your girlfriend. You have plenty of time to be engaged, be married, and have sex. I include sex because I have talked with several returned missionaries who feel that they rushed into marriage because they wanted to have sex. Take time to date many girls. If you find your soul mate on your very first date, at least do her the courtesy of dating a few other girls. If you don't, she won't be convinced that she is right for you. Sure, she might agree to marry you. But as soon as those tough times in marriage come, you will both start to question whether or not you really were meant for each other.

On your mission, you were used to praying all day, every day, about every decision you had to make. This is a very good habit to try and keep as long as you can. Pray about the girl that you want to be your girlfriend. Don't just ask, "Should she be my girlfriend?" Ask meaningful questions like, "Is this the person that I need to raise a family with? Will this person support me in all of my righteous endeavors in life and am I willing to support her? Does this person have all of the important qualities that I am searching for?" As you do this thoughtfully and prayerfully, you will know your answer.

As soon as you start dating someone for more than a couple dates, or as soon as you kiss, it is time for you to set up boundaries. A good place to start is in the "For the Strength of Youth" pamphlet. Talk with your significant other about your goals. Do you want to be clean enough to continue attending the temple? Do you want to be pure enough to remain as close to the Lord as you were on your mission? Meet with your bishop together and tell him about your boundaries and ask for his suggestions.

During this time, you will want to be together often. In so doing, you will find yourselves alone more frequently than before. Follow the boundaries that you have set for yourself as well as the suggestions given by your bishop or priesthood leader.

With Great Power Comes Great Responsibility

If your girlfriend hasn't served a mission, or even if she has, she may look to you as the more righteous part of your relationship. Just as you assume that your bishop who has been serving as a leader might have more knowledge or experience than one of your friends, she assumes that since you have dedicated two years of your life to serving the Lord that you will be more strong and righteous than she is. Do not abuse this respect she has for you. If you start to cross the line of immorality, she may justify that it must be ok because you (the returned missionary/priesthood holder) initiated it.

Engagement

"There is nothing unholy or degrading about sexuality in itself, for by that means men and women join in a process of creation and in an expression of love"
~Spencer W. Kimball

Once you are engaged, it is obvious that you both love each other very much and want to get married. You are getting more comfortable with each other both emotionally and physically. While this a very good and healthy thing, you must take extra caution not to go too far before marriage. Enough about this, you know the rules.

Each and every one of us here on this earth pride ourselves on being so unique and different from everyone else. Yet we also assume that everyone else believes and thinks exactly the same way that we do. I am always so surprised by how two people can fall in love and feel like they know each other so intimately, yet hardly know each other at all. Knowing your significant other's favorite color is nice, but doesn't help much when you are figuring out your finances.

I feel like there are several things that you should talk about with your significant other before you get too serious. I will include the major topics in this book, but for a complete list, please visit www.easypublishingcompany.com/marriage-questions. These are a few of the main topics that you should at least spend a few minutes discussing before getting married:

- Finances
- Children
- Life Goals
- Sex

As this is a book on intimacy, I will elaborate more on that last topic. Plan a date where you can get together and talk about sex. Try to find a private place where you won't be embarrassed to talk loud enough to each other, but also a place that you will be around other people. This gives you the privacy you will need without the opportunity to get too comfortable. A park would be a nice place.

Start off by talking about what you know about sex. What were you taught and how did you learn about it? Have you only had school maturation classes, friend's opinions, or parents that taught openly about sex? During this time and all times that you talk about sex, use the correct words and refrain from using any slang terms for body parts or other sex terms. Talk about your history with sex and encourage your significant other to talk about theirs. Be open and encouraging. Have you ever had any sexual experiences in your past? Has there been any sexual abuse or trauma? Has anything been done to deal with it?

When you feel like you have adequately covered both of your sexual histories, move on to concerns and preconceptions. Talk about what makes you or your significant other nervous about sex. Do you think it will hurt? Do you know what to do? What negative things have you heard about sex? How will you address and overcome these concerns together or separately? Are there any things that you don't think you would like to do? What things are you looking forward to sexually? What material would you both feel comfortable acquiring to learn more about sex and the many possibilities associated with it?

At this time, you might be wondering what things you should share with your partner about your past. Because of the seriousness that the Lord has placed on the Law of Chastity, sexual transgression is not something that we can talk about easily. I would recommend talking to your bishop about what you should or shouldn't tell your significant other. However, a good rule of thumb is the following: Would you want to know about this sexual experience if it were something in your partner's past? If so, you should definitely have a talk. Another idea is to ask what things your partner would like to know about form your past.

One book that I would highly recommend to anyone, especially those that aren't very comfortable with sex is *And they were not Ashamed* by Laura M. Brotherson. This book was written by a BYU professor who has had years of experience with marriage and sexual counseling. It is written more for girls, but is very informative for men. This book goes over the role of sex in marriage and how important it is in God's plan for each of us. It has important sections on past trauma and dealing with negative feelings toward sex.

At this time, talk about your turn-ons and turn-offs. You might not know everything, because most of you haven't had sex yet. But think about when you have kissed or even made out. Does bad breath turn you off? Do you think that seeing a lot of pubic hair might turn you off? What outfits do you and your partner find appealing? Talk about everything and anything that you are looking forward to.

If you are a girl, make sure you see your gynecologist before you get married. Both of you make sure that you are looking your best. Figure out if you want to use birth control and which kind. You want to be clean and free of any odors. Buy some items that might help you out on your honeymoon. Some suggestions are lubricant, condoms, and oils. Anything that you are comfortable with is a good idea.

Honeymoon Night

"They were both naked, the man and his wife, and were not ashamed."
~Genesis 2:24

Unfortunately, the honeymoon night and the next few nights can lay the foundation for a healthy or unhealthy sexual relationship. Men, for some reason, have been created with the ability to have orgasms much easier than women. Because of this, many men screw up their wife's sexual experience. If men only think of themselves, they can make their wife hate sex forever. Do not be nervous; just be sure that you aren't selfish. Let me try to explain this a little bit better.

When a man puts his penis in a girl's vagina for vaginal intercourse, his penis must be erect. For his penis to be erect, he must be sexually aroused. A man must be aroused in order to participate in sex. Most men orgasm very quickly compared to women. A girl does not have to be aroused to participate in sex. Some women go through their entire life having sex without enjoying it. This would be comparable to having sex with your partner without getting an erection. Or maybe just as you are getting an erection, your partner orgasms, rolls over, and falls quickly asleep.

Your entire goal for your honeymoon should be to bring pleasure to your partner, whether that results in orgasm or not. For a girl to have an orgasm, she must be relaxed, aroused, and have an adequate amount of time. You will need to figure out how to achieve all of these things with your partner, as every person is very different. Next, I will give you an example rundown for your honeymoon night.

Much, if not most, of a woman's arousal is emotional. This means that most women need a lot of emotional arousal before any sexual arousal can happen. After the wedding on your way to the hotel, talk about your feelings. Tell your new spouse how excited you are to be with her. Tell her how much you love her and how you are anticipating an amazing life together. As most girls are much more nervous about sex than men, do not talk strictly about sex. Talk about the honeymoon ahead of you and the feelings you felt as you got married earlier in the day.

When you get to the hotel room, do everything you can to create a calm, stress-free environment. Suggest taking a shower (either separately or together) to wash off the smells and stresses of the day. Offer to give your partner a massage before you get started. Take at least 10-15 minutes massaging your partner. Do not go straight for the vagina or breasts. Finish the massage with her wanting you to touch her there. Be very gentle and unrushed.

Next, without making your partner feel like you have a set schedule, begin foreplay. Go from massaging her back, arms, and feet to gently kissing her neck and lips. Kiss and enjoy each other for several minutes. Then begin to take off your partner's clothes. From now on, begin whispering things to your partner about how much you love her or how attracted you are to her. While you are kissing, touch her ENTIRE body. Again, do not go straight for the breasts or vagina. Touch her everywhere, but those places. Get close to these sensitive areas but go around them. Once you have touched her entire body, you can go to her breasts and vagina.

While continuing to kiss and fondle each other, begin to rub your partner's clitoris (image to follow). The clitoris is at the very top of the opening of the vagina. Be very gentle and do this for a while. Every girl is different, but make sure to give sufficient stimulation to the clitoris before entering the vagina. For most women, this is anywhere from 5-20 minutes. Your goal is to get her sexually aroused. Talk to her and ask her what she likes and what feels good.

Once she has been sufficiently aroused (or climaxed), apply lubricant to your penis and slowly, gently enter her vagina. If this causes too much pain, pull back out and enter part way. Try entering one or two fingers to stretch the vagina. What ever you do, do not put your partner through pain just so you can enjoy yourself.

This has all been a simple example of what might work for you and your partner. I want to share with you an example that I hear all too often from girl's about their honeymoon night:

You get back to your hotel room and she puts on some lingerie. You are so excited to finally have sex that you rip off the lingerie, put your penis in her vagina, and climax. Then you roll over and fall asleep. I want to assume that this happens because of lack of knowledge of female sexuality and NOT because a man is just trying to fulfill his selfish desires. If you do not pay adequate attention to your wife and her pleasure and arousal, you can easily turn her off to sex for the rest of your marriage.

The biggest tip I can give anyone that is about to get married is to pay attention to their spouse and his or her needs. Do anything that you are comfortable with that makes them feel special and loved. Be open and loving with your spouse and tell him or her what feels good and what you like or don't like.

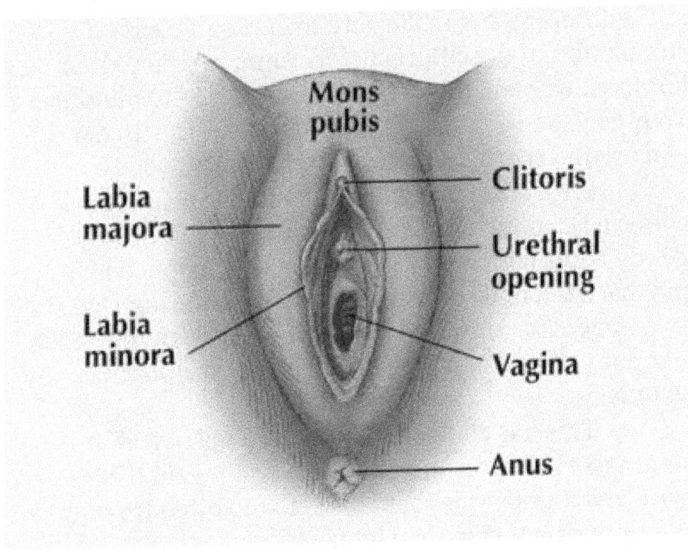

This simple diagram of a vagina is only meant to help you with your sexual understanding. The vagina is the opening between a girl's legs where a man can insert his penis during vaginal intercourse. The clitoris is the sensitive spot for females. In order for them to achieve an orgasm, most of the stimulation will usually occur here.

Sex life in marriage

"Married couples should also understand that sexual relations within marriage are divinely approved not only for the purpose of procreation, but also as a way of expressing love and strengthening emotional and spiritual bonds between husband and wife."

~First Presidency, The Church Handbook of Instructions, section 21.4.4

Intimacy in marriage is a very important matter. Because most men feel love through physical intimacy, an unhealthy sex life can ruin an otherwise healthy relationship between husband and wife. The very best way to ensure a success in your own marriage is to include a 3rd person. As long as you, your spouse, and your Heavenly Father have an equal role in your relationship, you will be able to successfully traverse your way through many of life's trials and difficulties.

There are several books available that talk more about intimacy within marriage. I wanted mainly to focus on how to achieve healthy intimacy right after you return from serving a mission. Therefore, I will end with one last part. The LDS church has been very vague and somewhat confusing when it comes to what is appropriate after marriage. While many people find this frustrating, I understand where they are coming from. If they were to issue a document stating everything within marriage that is ok and everything that isn't ok, they would be opening up a Pandora's Box of problems.

There would most definitely be those people that need the letter of the law spelled out. They would claim, "The church said I couldn't have sex with horses, but it said NOTHING about cows." I am not trying to be vulgar or make light of this topic, but just trying to illustrate how ridiculous things would get. The First Presidency would be getting letters daily of church members asking about new positions, new sex acts, etc. Below I am going to answer the most common questions I've heard as best as I can.

How often should a couple have sex?

This typically translates to, "One of us wants more sex and one of us wants less sex." If both of you want to have sex more frequently, you should have sex more frequently. If both of you want to limit the sexual experiences you are having together, then it will be easy to reduce them. The problem is when there are different desires for sex (which is pretty much present in every relationship.) When this is the case, you need to determine what is making one partner want less sex? Everything about intimacy in marriage requires openness and understanding. If you can't have this talk with just the two of you, go see a marriage counselor.

Both the husband and wife need to be understanding of one another's needs. The short answer to this question is, "You should have sex as much as both of you want it. It doesn't depend on the national average. It doesn't depend on just one of you. You need to come to some agreement that both of you are happy with." If both of you have a different answer to this question, it definitely needs to be discussed soon. One, or both, partners in a marriage left feeling unsatisfied or unfulfilled can lead to very negative consequences.

What is ok to do in the Bedroom?

Believe me, I wish that there were a simple answer to this just as much as you do. You will find that many people don't know the answer. Many people feel like they are experts on this question and will give you very different answers. Many people will even cite church leaders or documents with seemingly opposing views. There are a few parts to this question. First, if one of you is uncomfortable doing anything in the bedroom, neither of you should participate in it.

That doesn't mean that it's unacceptable forever, but it is unacceptable while one of you is feeling uncomfortable. You should never force your spouse to engage in any sexual act that he or she is uncomfortable with. This could be something as harmless as traditional vaginal intercourse. The point is, sex is such a sacred and fragile act that you should not do anything that will make your spouse think of you, or trust you, less.

A statement offered by the first presidency stated that a couple should not participate in anything that is *"unnatural, impure, or unholy"* sexually. Like I said earlier, there are so many people with differing views on what is unnatural that this statement doesn't clear much up. I am not an official spokesperson of the church and I am not saying that the following is how every church member should believe. However, let me offer up a few suggestions.

First, every single one of us is entitled to personal revelation. That means that if we are living a righteous life and have pure desires, our Heavenly Father will let us know if something isn't right by way of the Holy Ghost. Second, a husband and wife as a couple are entitled to receive revelation for their marriage and their family. This means that, as a couple, you are also entitled to receive an answer together.

I know that my wording needs to be very careful for this next statement. Let me start by saying that I sustain all church leaders to receive revelation for their corresponding roles. We are all human and sometimes humans will make mistakes even when they have the best of intentions. Sometimes when couples go to a bishop, that bishop will share with the couple what HE thinks is right. He is sharing what HE thinks is the interpretation of "unnatural, impure, or unholy", and what is most likely the revelation that he and his wife have received in their marriage. That doesn't mean that what he says is necessarily right for your marriage. I would personally leave the bishop as a last resort for this specific topic. If you and your spouse can feel comfortable and worthy with the sexual things that both of you would like to participate in, then there is no need to get further guidance.

Is it ok to view pornography if it is done together?

Absolutely not. The church has taken a very strict stance on pornography, cautioning members to "avoid it at all costs." Pornography is very destructive to families and relationships. If one or both partners start to view pornography, it is imperative that you both support one another to get this issue resolved. Do not keep it in the dark. Tell your spouse. Tell your bishop. Tell your family. Pornography flourishes in the dark and the only way to break free is to bring it into the light. There are several books on the subject of pornography, so I will leave it at that.

Easy Publishing Company